This book belongs to: _____

Draw a picture of yourself/s

http://www.fast-print.net/bookshop

SOUNDTRACK TO MY LIFE
Copyright © John Osborne 2106

All rights reserved

No part of this book may be reproduced in any form by photocopying or any electronic or mechanical means, including information storage or retrieval systems, without permission in writing from both the copyright owner and the publisher of the book.

The right of John Osborne to be identified as the authors of this work has been asserted by him in accordance with the Copyright, Design and Patents Act 1988 and any subsequent amendments thereto.

A catalogue record for this book is available from the British Library

ISBN 978-178456-425-4

First published 2016 by Fast-Print Publishing, Peterborough, England.

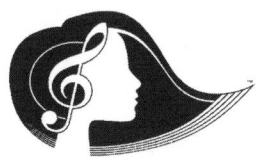

Soundtrack to My Life

For Maisie and Roy

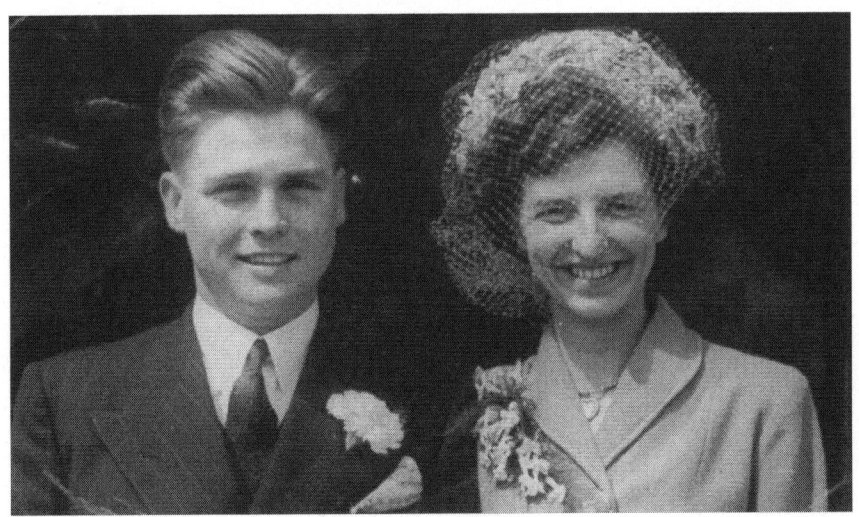

"Joy, sorrow, lamentation, laughter - to all these
music gives voice, but in such a way
that we are transported from the world
of unrest to a world of peace"

Albert Schweitzer

Contents

Foreword	Page 7
Soundtrack to My Life Core Principles	Page 8
Why Music?	Page 9
Using The Book	Page 11
My Family	Page 14
My Favourites	Page 20
My Events	Page 26
My Romance	Page 32
My Feelings	Page 38
My Future	Page 44
My Dislikes	Page 50
My Soundtrack to My Life Playlist	Page 52
Practical Application of 'Soundtrack to My Life'	Page 53
Technology	Page 54
Existing Collections	Page 55
Choosing the Right Device	Page 55

Acknowledgements

This book would not have been possible without the involvement of two remarkable women **Kate Williams** and **Farai Pfende**. Together we make up the Joco Team. They have worked tirelessly with me to develop the ideas, resources and courses that make up our **'Music in Care'** programme. Their belief in what we do, their passion, professionalism, creativity and ability to take my muddled ramblings and turn them into beautiful images and meaningful text is truly awesome.

Kate Fisher for her enthusiasm, support and belief in what we do

Tom Kitwood for his inspirational model of psychological wellbeing and personhood.

musicworks for their support and assistance in developing this project.

Foreword

Living with dementia, or caring for someone with dementia, requires attention to not only physical needs but also meaningful engagement and interaction. No doubt it can be challenging but, as a carer for my father who had dementia, I found that the time spent with him was always better when we tried to enter his reality. When we took time to understand where he was and what mattered to him most, he was more relaxed, humorous and engaged. Conversation became lively and at times hilarious, peppered with recollections and memories of shared experiences. The pressure was off and Roy was 'Roy the person' not just 'Roy the dementia'.

This book arose out of my personal and professional care experiences and a desire to help people to find a positive way to reach and connect with people living with dementia that focuses on strengths, ability and joy. Through my musical and care knowledge I developed this book with a variety of music questions that draw on life stories, generate positive and meaningful conversations, trigger reconnections to the past and promote a person's sense of self. The resulting personalised playlists of their significant music can be used on a day-to-day basis to enhance quality of life and promote emotional and spiritual wellbeing.

Recognition of the value of this approach came in 2012 with a national award for innovation in care. Later, research undertaken at the Institute of Mental Health in Nottingham, supported the value of **'Soundtrack'** to both people with dementia and those who cared for them.

I created **Joco Learning and Development** to provide person centred training for health and social care staff in the application of **'Music in Care'**. Professional carers, family carers and musicians have all benefitted from the training and the therapeutic application of music.

The **'Soundtrack to My Life'** book will hopefully take you on an enjoyable journey down your musical memory lane and bring enrichment and flourishing to those living with dementia and their loved ones.

Here's to living well with dementia!

Soundtrack to My Life Core Principles

These are the values that underpin **'Soundtrack to My Life'**. I ask you to bear them in mind as you complete this book.

- People with dementia do not lose the ability to communicate, we lose the ability to understand them.

- You cannot work with people with dementia without knowing their life history.

- We are all capable of using music to create memory bridges and reconnections that support people with dementia to live well.

Why Music?

Music is strongly linked to life events and experiences that define who we are. Music can transport us to a particular time or place and release strong emotions. It can calm and soothe us or motivate us and help us to find energy and drive. Music can greatly improve the quality of our lives.

In people living with dementia it has been shown to have the following benefits:

- Enhance well-being

- Reduce stress

- Promote relaxation

- Enhance cognitive function and memory

- Improve communication

- Express feelings

- Reconnect to memories and relationships

- Assist with physical rehabilitation

Music can provoke an emotional response even if you have never heard it before. However, if you choose to listen to music which is significant to you personally you should experience the benefits listed in abundance. This is why the **'Soundtrack to My Life'** toolkit was created.

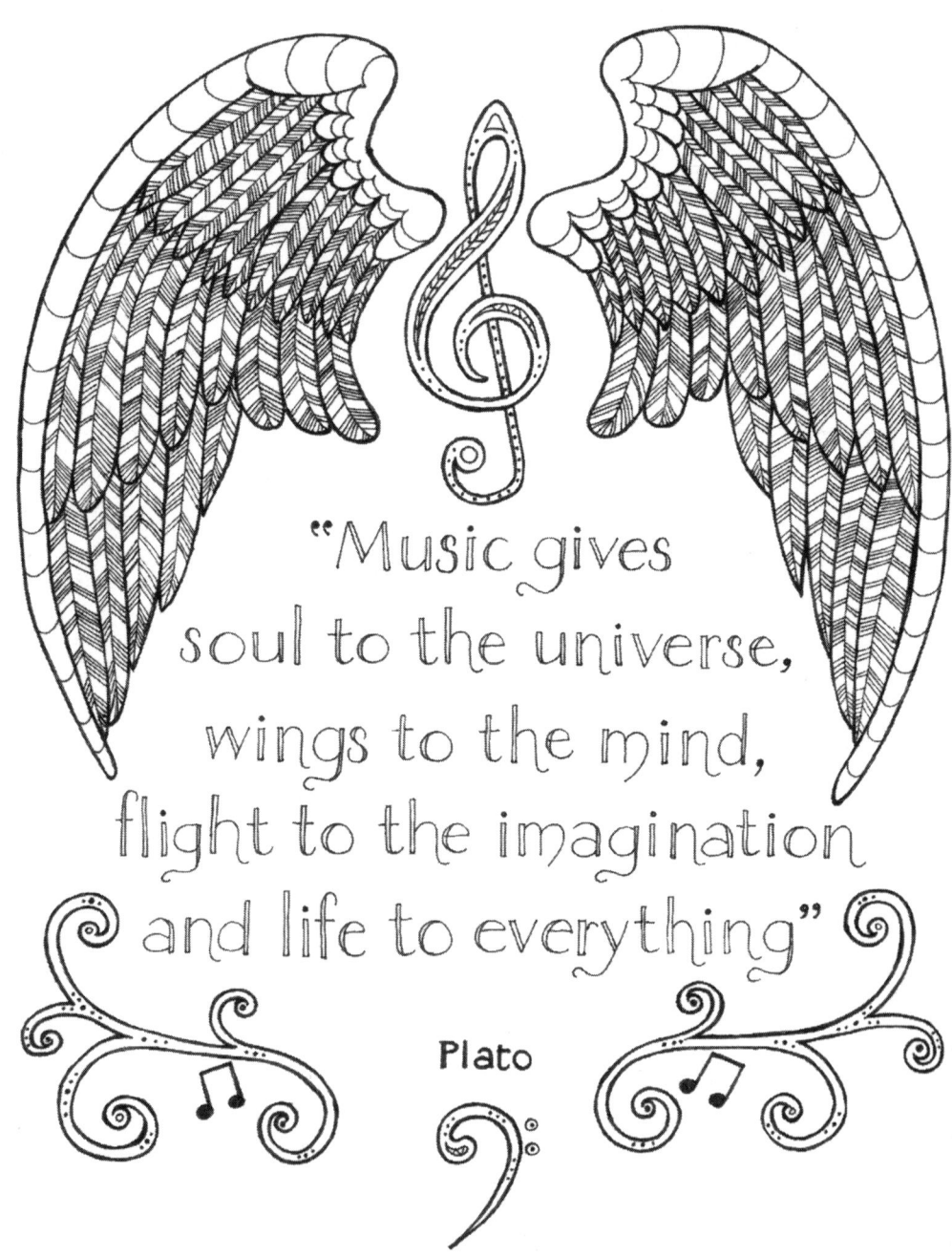

Using the Book

The book has been designed in such a way that it can be carried around with you and used by yourself and others whenever it will be helpful to do so.

Choosing the music that is most significant to you and recording the reasons for your choices provides a rich resource for you and others to use to enhance daily living and life experiences.

It will help you to remain connected to your sense of self, your past and those who mean most to you.

REMEMBER!
- Take your time - enjoy!

- Don't be over-influenced by what other people think - this is YOUR **'Soundtrack'**

- Involve people close to you to help recall memories and events if you wish

- There are no right or wrong answers! Please use the questions in the book as you wish. For example, if a question isn't relevant to you, leave it blank or if you have three favourite singers rather than one, record all three.

Recording

The questions within the **'Soundtrack to My Life'** are designed to prompt you to think about people, events and feelings that may be important to you. Some questions may not be relevant to you and you may wish to leave them blank.

In the space provided under each question, record the piece(s) of music including the artist(s) if that is significant. For example you may like 'Yesterday' by the Beatles but prefer a version recorded by Frank Sinatra.

It is important that you record the story of why that piece of music is important to you and the memories linked to it. Was it playing when you met your partner? Did you sing it with your family? Was it something you sang at church or school as a child?

Dislikes

You will find there is a section entitled **'Dislikes'** for you to record the music and sounds that you really don't want to hear. There is obviously no favourites section on this page and you do not need to include anything from this section on your **'Playlist'** page.

Activities

Throughout the book, spaces have been left for you to record your thoughts, feelings, frustrations, hopes and fears. There are activities that you can undertake if you wish. For example, there are drawings that can be coloured in or left blank, spaces where sketches or pictures can be inserted. Just find your creativity as encouraged by the music choices you have made.

Did you know?
6 amazing facts about music and how it affects your brain:
1. Your heartbeat changes to mimic the music you are listening to - this also affects blood pressure and breathing
2. A song you can't seem to get out of your head is called an "earworm"
3. If you get "chills" when you listen to music, this is mostly caused by the release of Dopamine, the "pleasure chemical" while anticipating the peak moment of the song
4. Learning a musical instrument can improve fine motor and reasoning skills
5. Music is one of the few activities in life that utilises the entire brain.
6. Playing music regularly can physically alter your brain structure

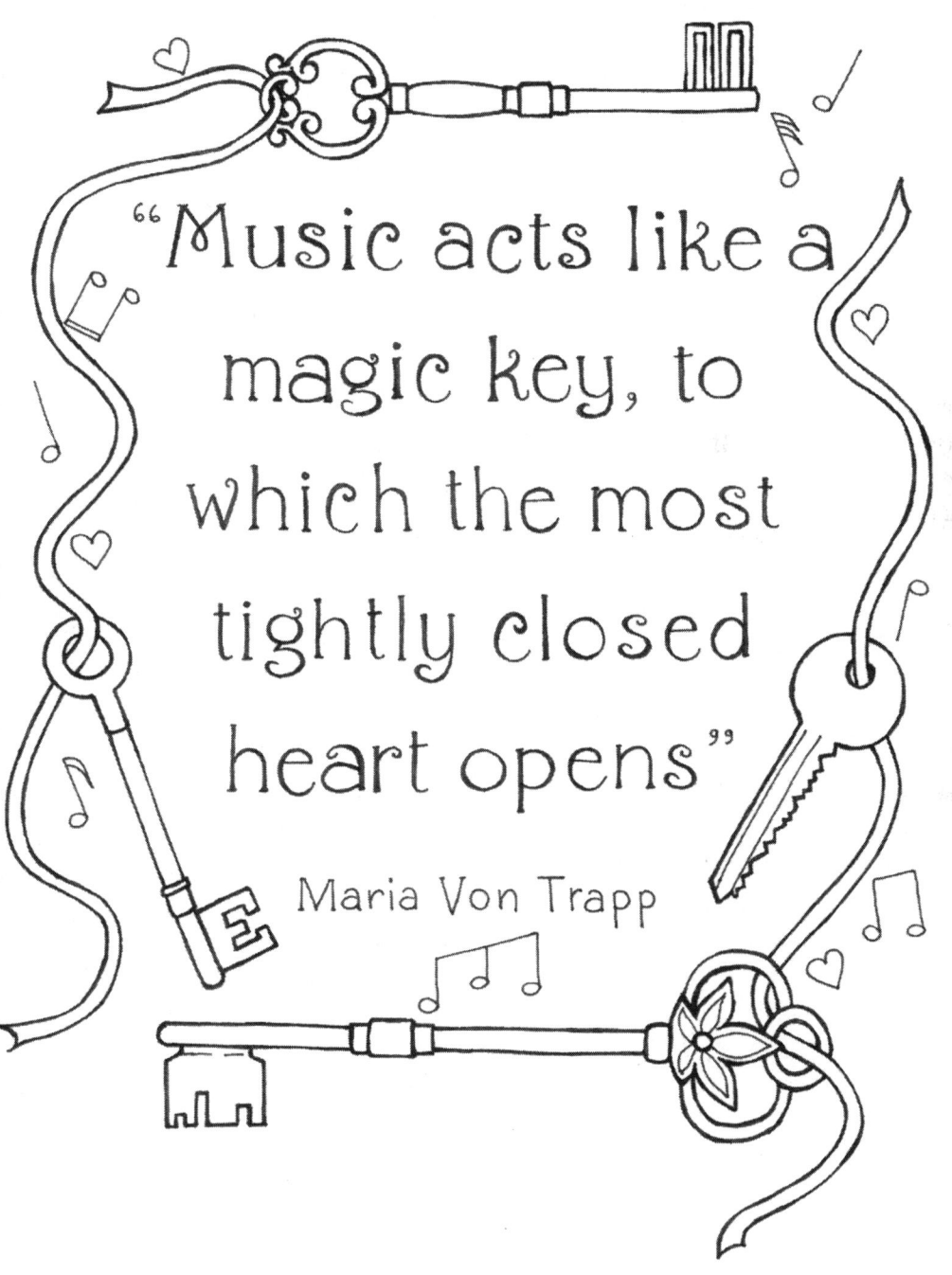

MY FAMILY

Music that reminds me of my children

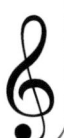

Music that reminds me of my family

Music that reminds me of my Mum

Music that reminds me of my Dad

Draw or stick in pictures of your Mum, Dad, children or other family members you want to include.

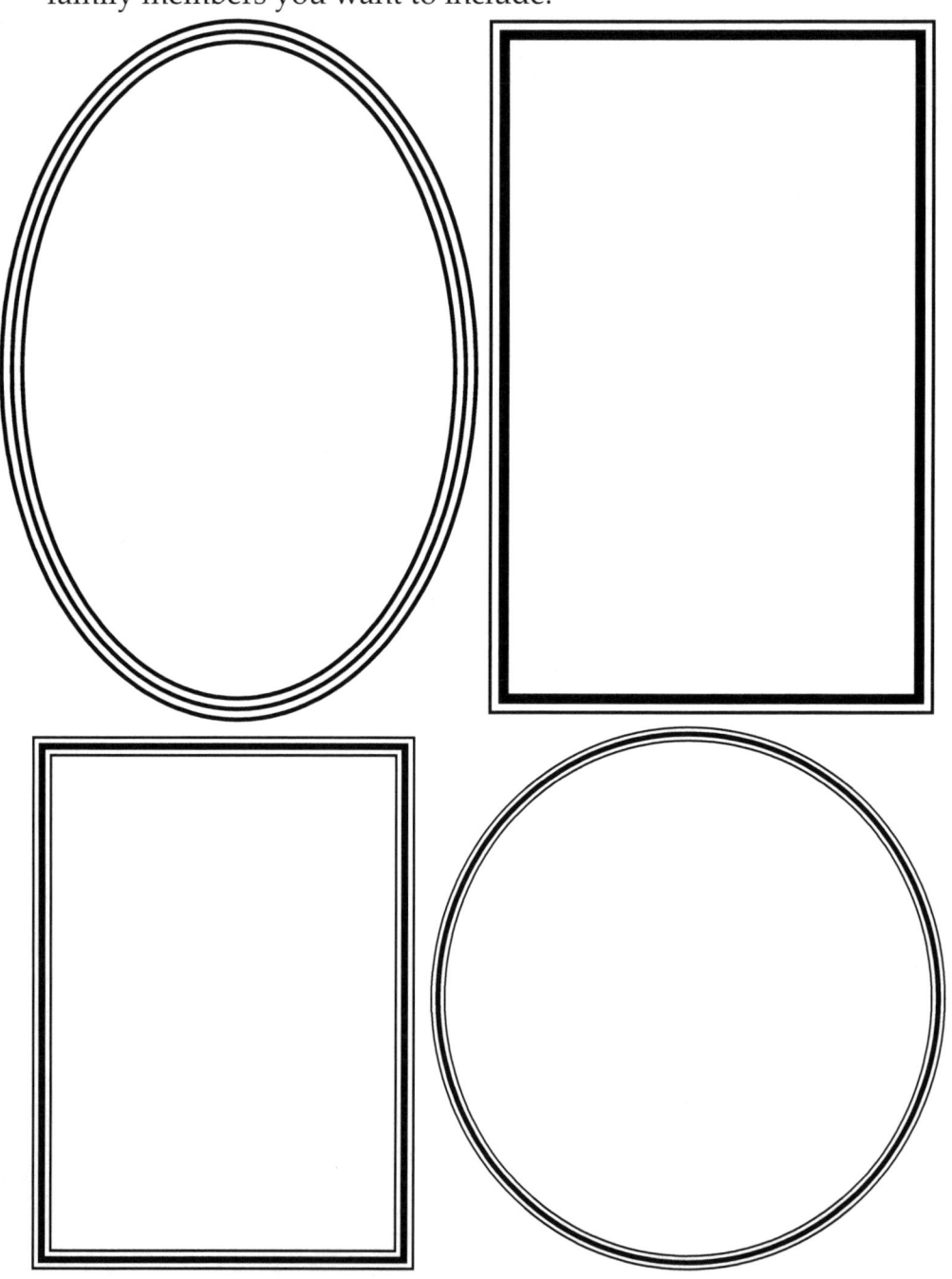

Music that reminds me of my childhood

Music that reminds me of someone I have lost

MEMORY PAGE: Use this page to record special family memories

My two favourites from 'MY FAMILY' are:

1.

2.

Add these to your playlist on Page 52

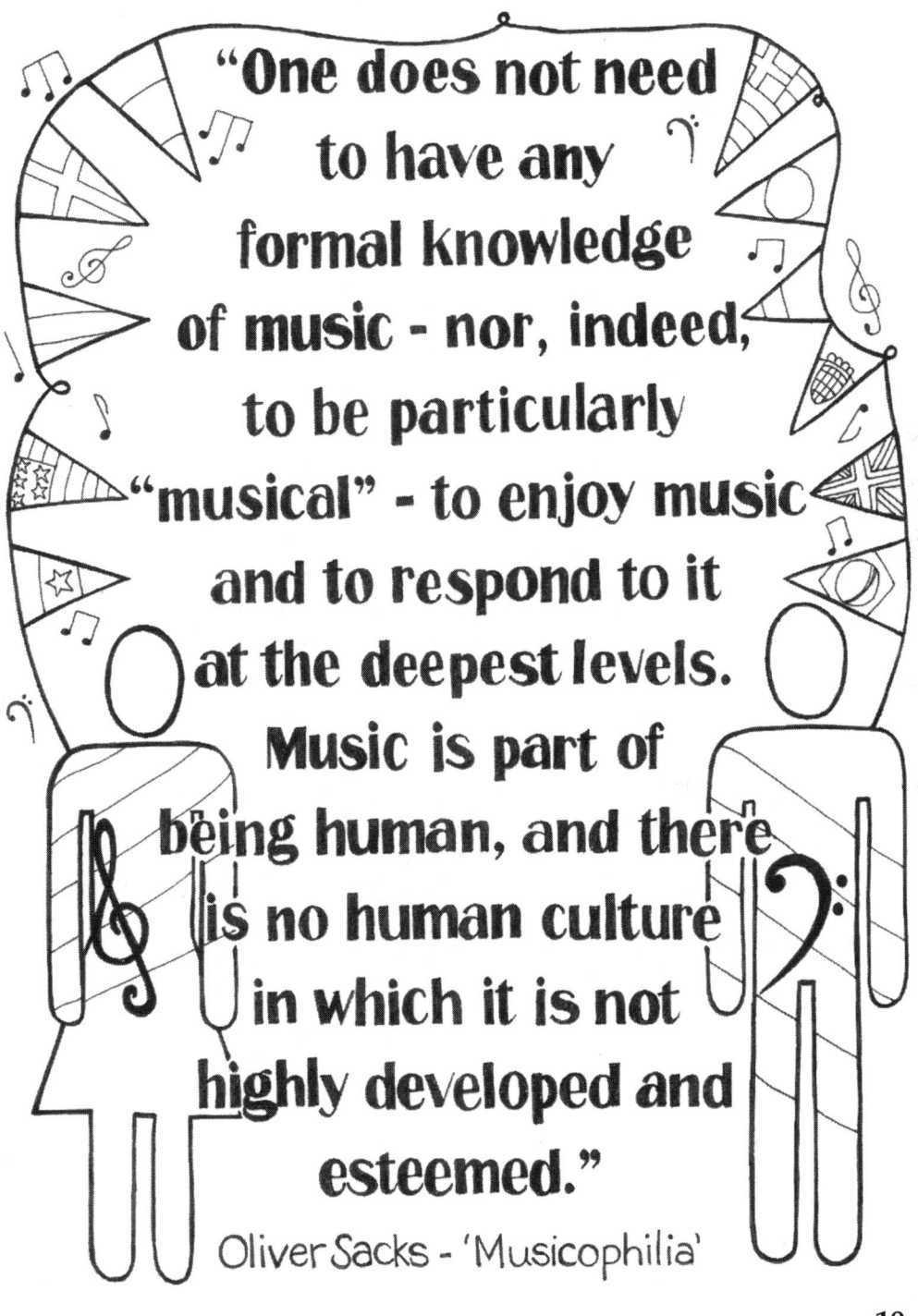

MY FAVOURITES

My favourite song or piece of music

My favourite singer or musician

My favourite song to sing along to

Fill this thought bubble with pictures, words, drawings or memories that remind you of your musical guilty pleasures.

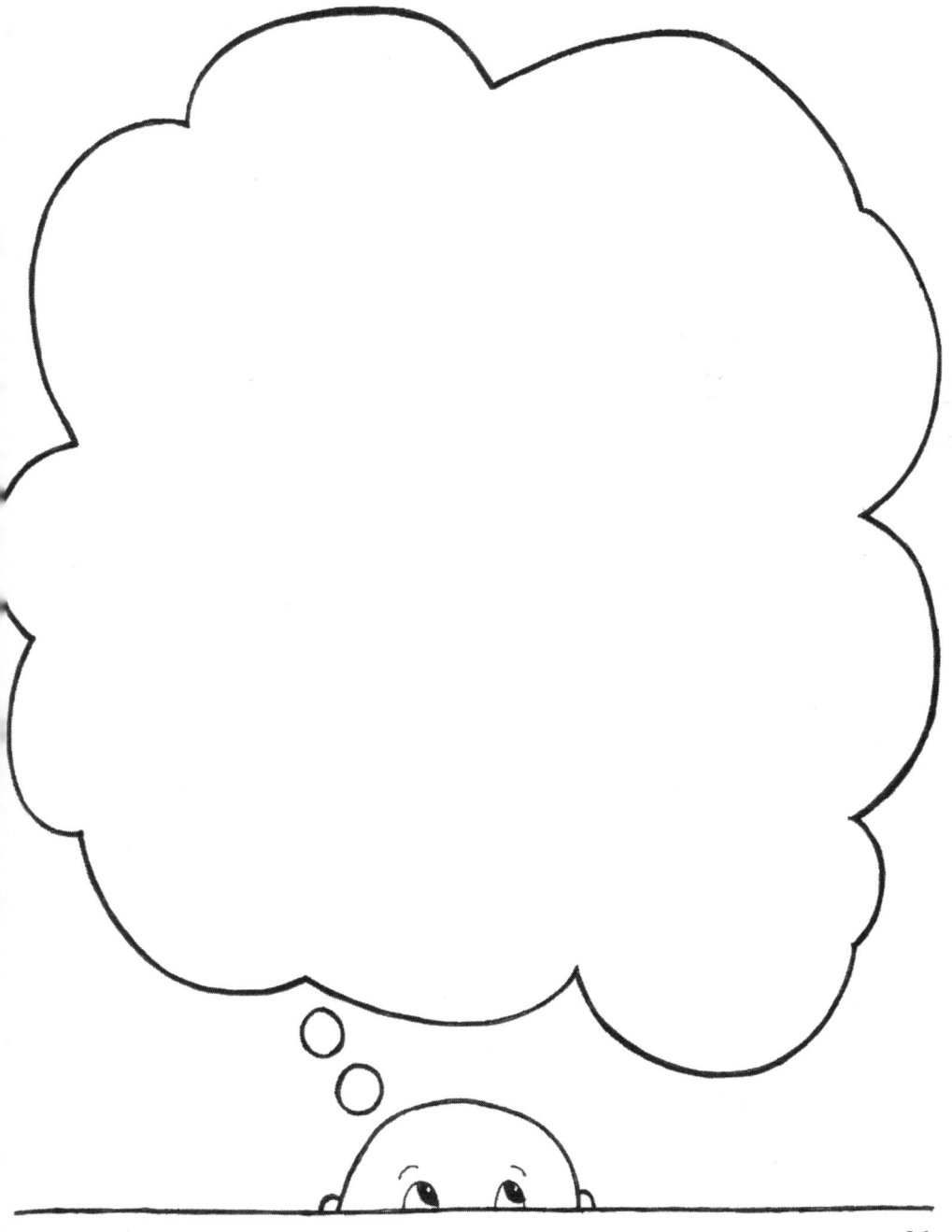

My favourite piece of religious or spiritual music

My favourite music to relax to

My favourite music to celebrate to

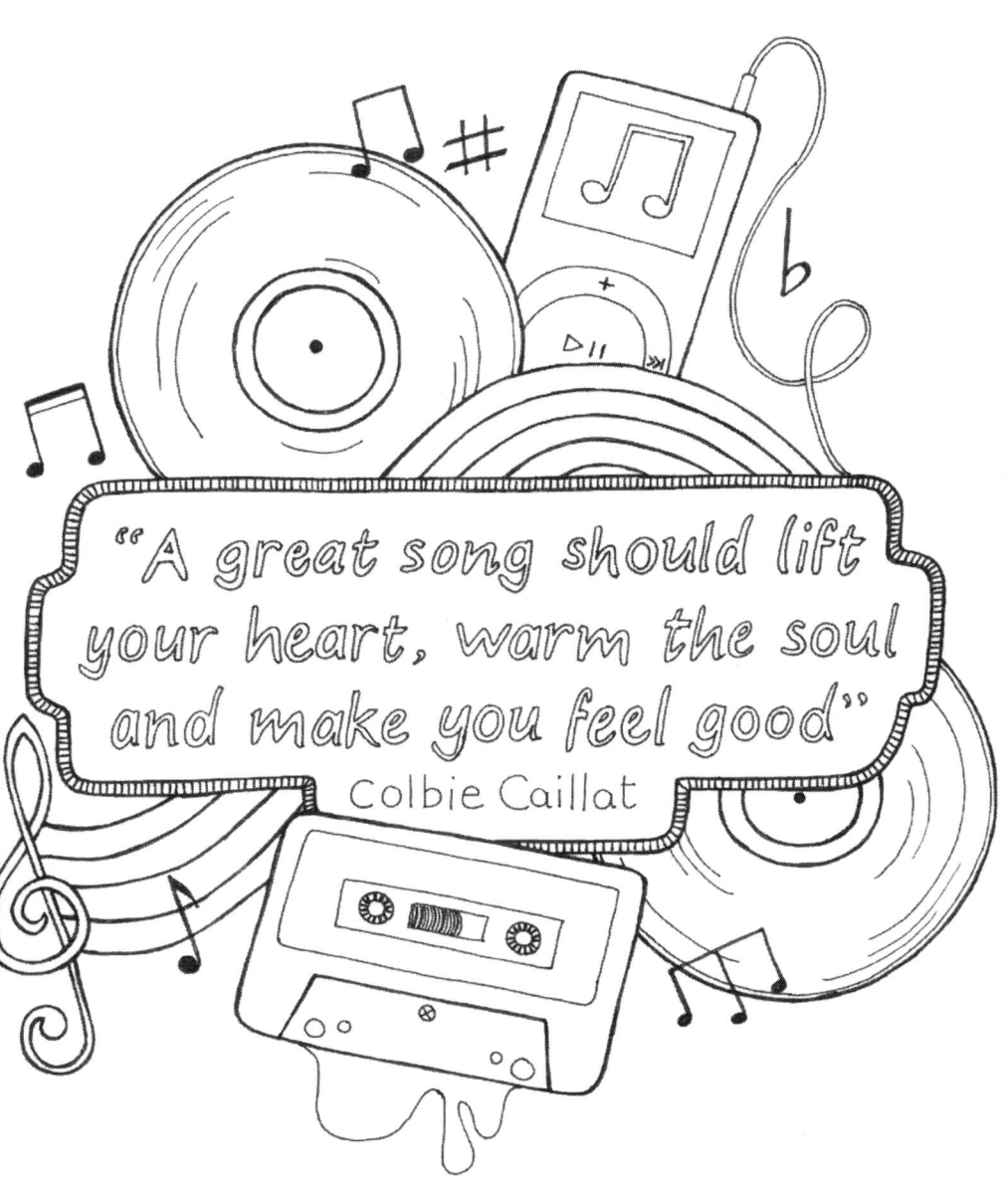

Favourite music to share with others

Favourite music to listen to alone

MEMORY PAGE: Use this page to record memories of good times with your favourite music or musicians

My two favourites from 'MY FAVOURITES' are:

1.

2.

Add these to your playlist on Page 52

MY EVENTS

Music of my culture

My favourite sports music

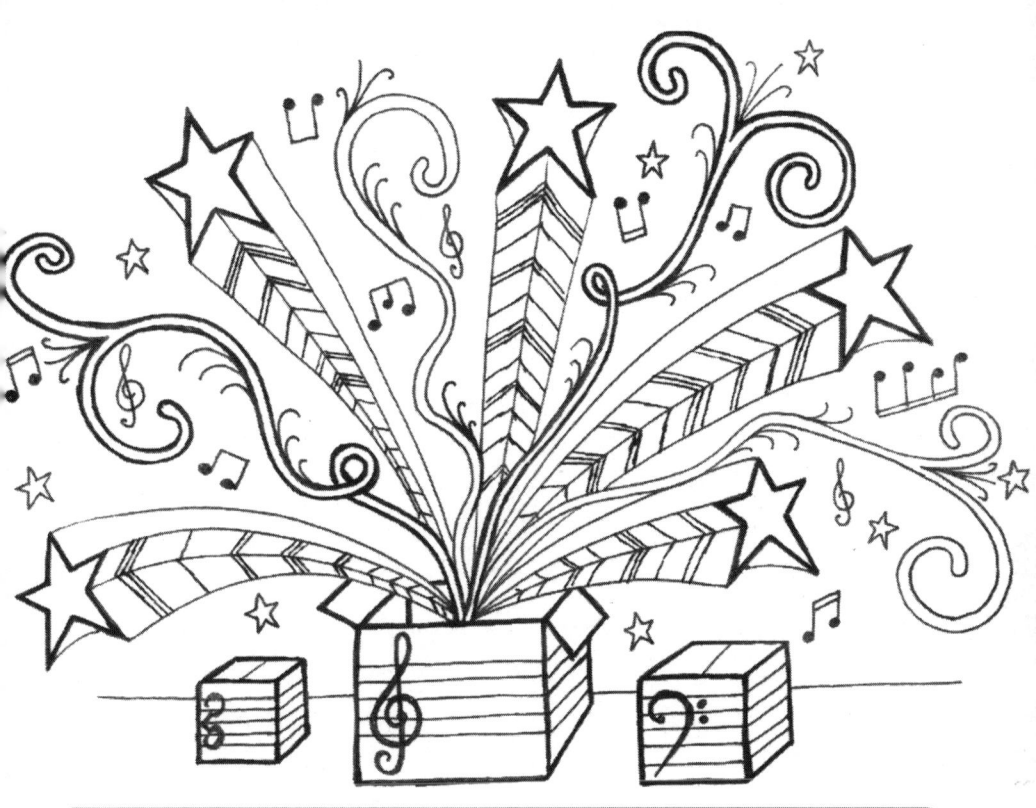

Music that reminds me of my holidays

Music that reminds me of my wedding

Music that reminds me of a special meeting

"I've found that no matter what life throws at me, music softens the blow."

Bryce Anderson

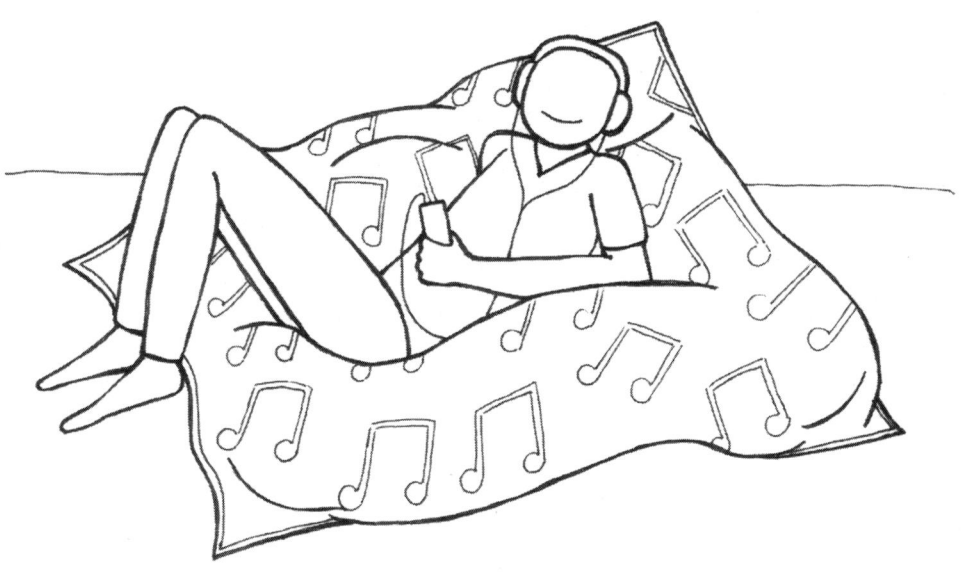

My favourite music festival

My favourite music from a concert or performance

MEMORY PAGE: Use this page to record memories of special events, shows, concerts and festivals you have been to.

My two favourites from 'MY EVENTS' are:

1.

2.

Add these to your playlist on Page 52

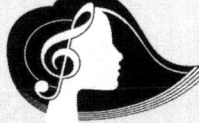

MY ROMANCE

Music that reminds me of my partner

Music that reminds me of when I first met my partner

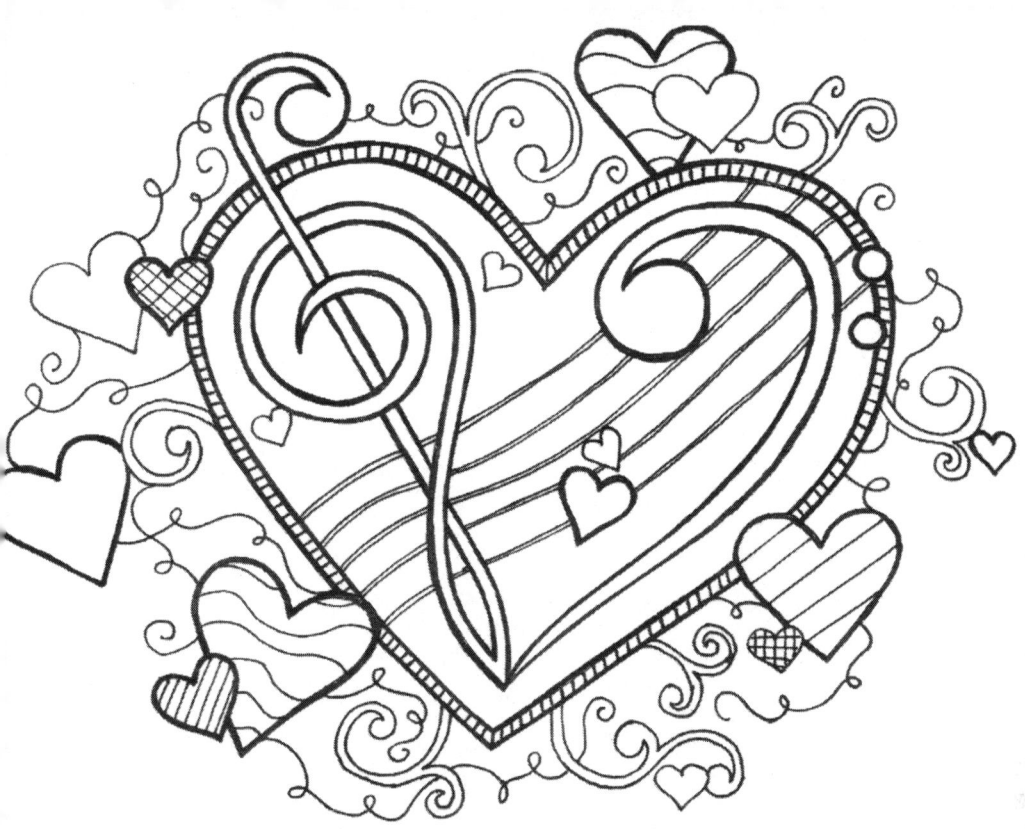

My favourite love song

Music that makes me feel 'in love'

Did you know?

According to *about.com* the top 10 greatest love songs are:

10. "I Got You Babe" - *Sonny & Cher* (1965)
9. "And I Love Her" - *The Beatles* (1964)
8. "In Your Eyes" - *Peter Gabriel* (1986)
7. "Unchained Melody" - *Righteous Brothers* (1965)
6. "Your Song" - *Elton John* (1970)
5. "Wonderful Tonight" - *Eric Clapton* (1978)
4. "Just The Way You Are" - *Billy Joel* (1977)
3. "Maybe I'm Amazed" - *Paul McCartney* (1977)
2. "The First Time Ever I Saw Your Face" - *Roberta Flack* (1972)
1. "Something" - *The Beatles* (1969)

Music that reminds me of a childhood sweetheart

Music that got me through "break-ups"

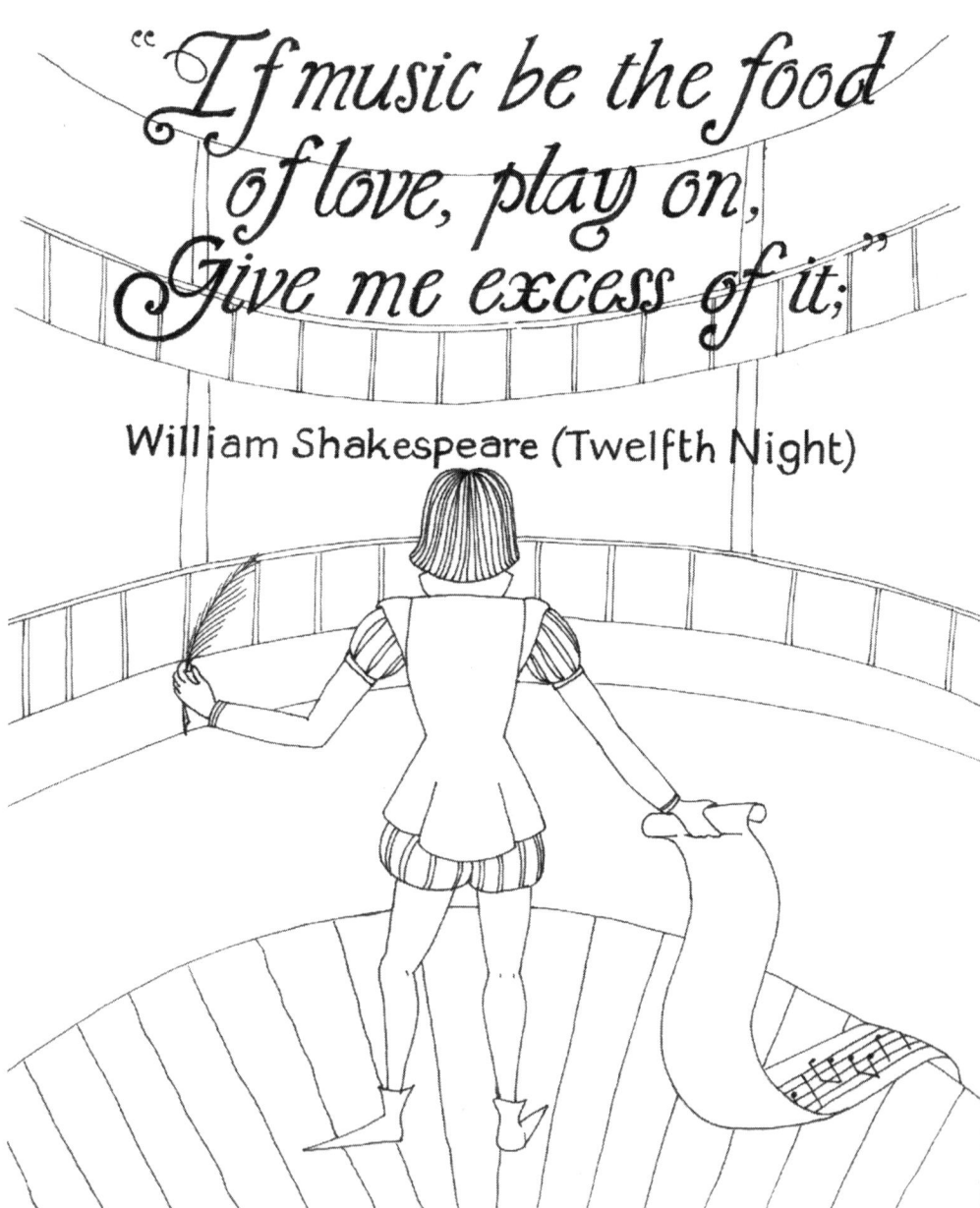

MEMORY PAGE: Use this page to record memories of musical romantic moments

My two favourites from 'MY ROMANCE' are:

1.

2.

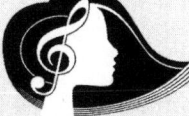

Add these to your playlist on Page 52

MY FEELINGS

Music that makes me feel like dancing

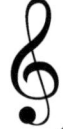

Music that makes me feel like singing

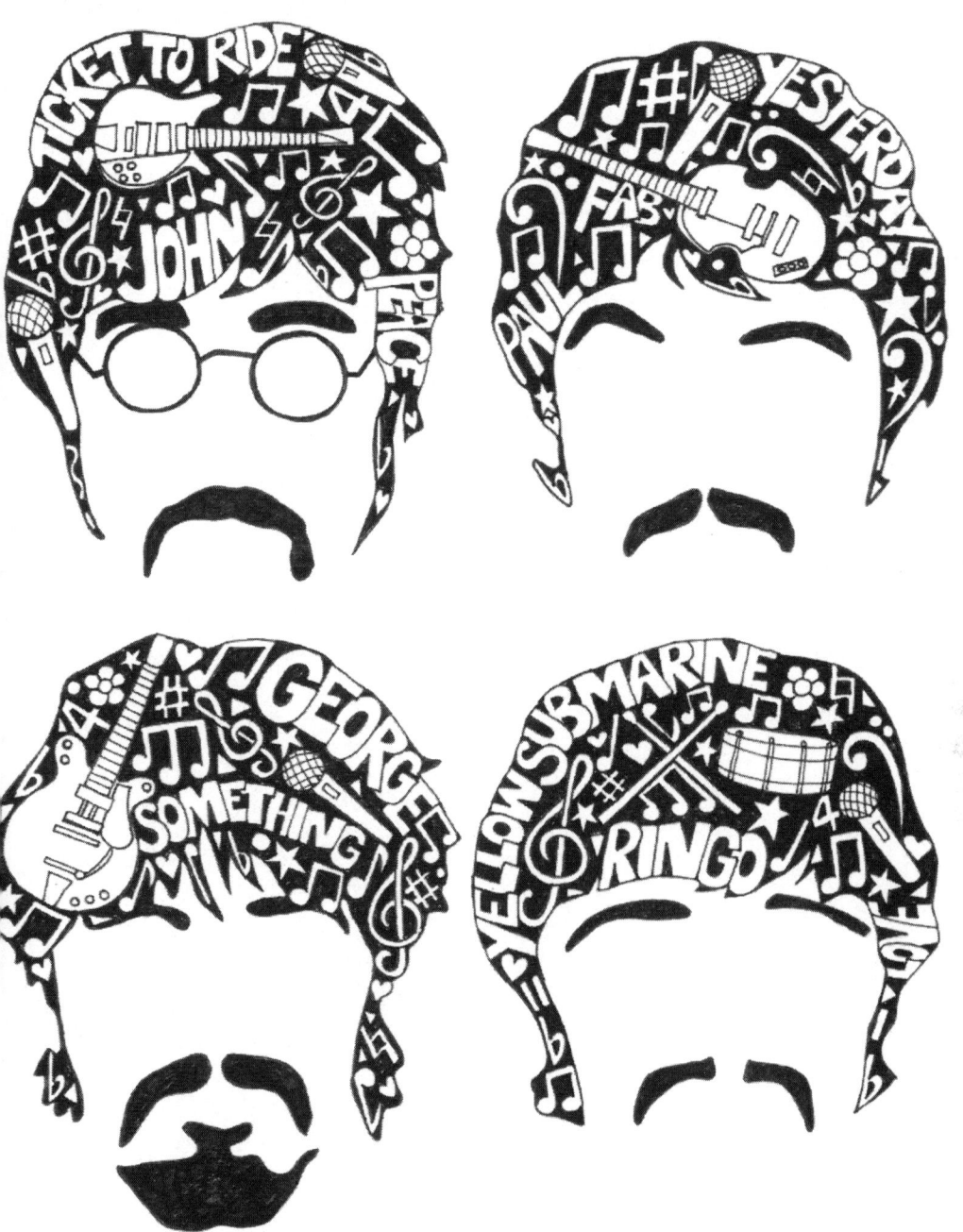

Music that makes me feel happy

Music that makes me feel sad

Music that came from my best time/era

Music that makes me feel calm and relaxed

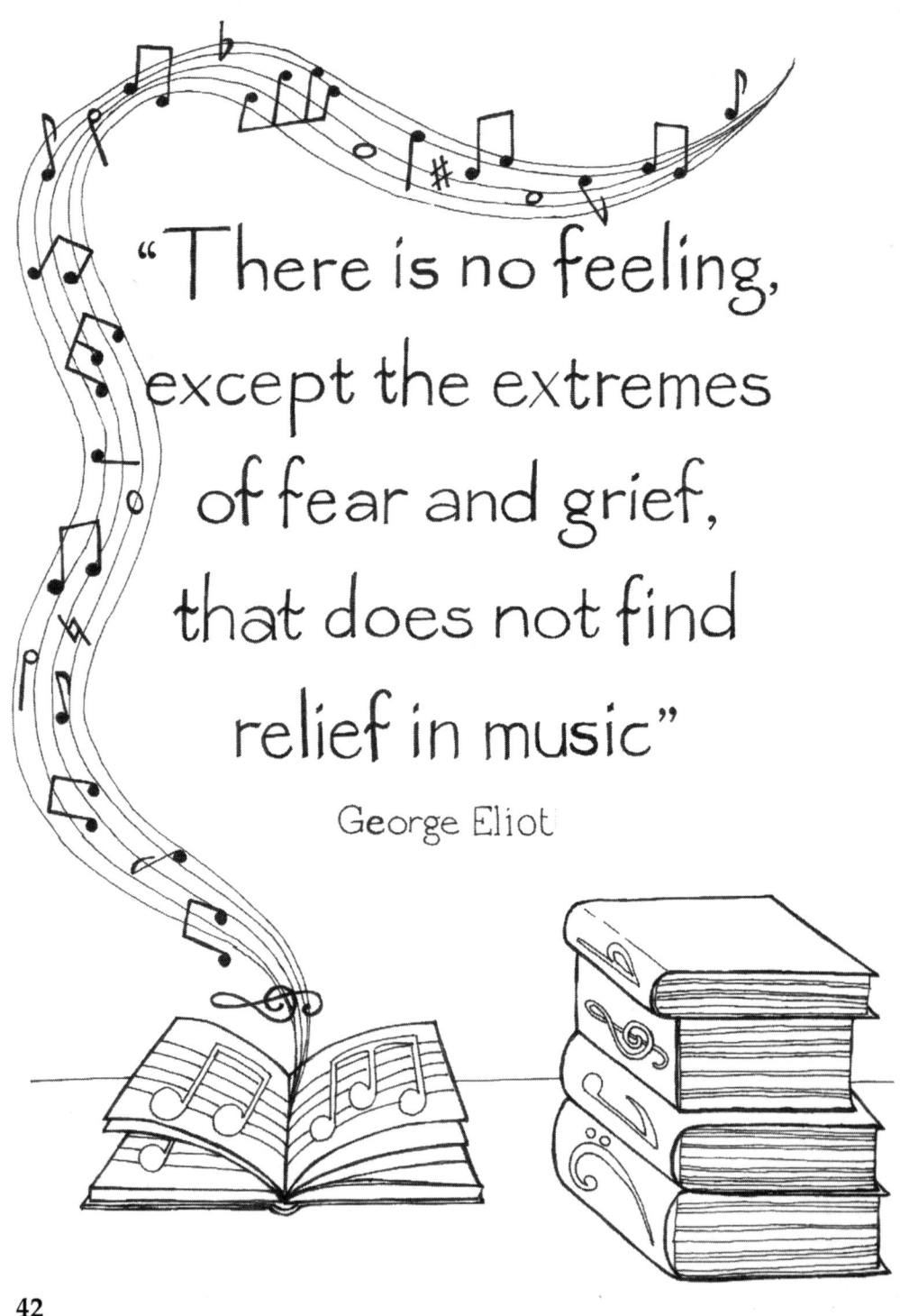

MEMORY PAGE: Use this page to record memories of people, things, activities and places that make you feel positive.

My two favourites from 'MY FEELINGS' are:

1.

2.

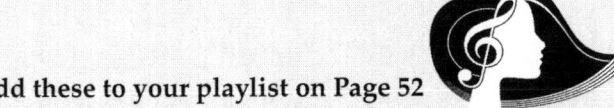

Add these to your playlist on Page 52

MY FUTURE

Music to get up to

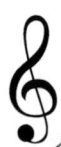

Music to go to bed to

My Musical Bucket List

Who are the performers you would like to see, songs you'd like to hear, instruments you'd like to try or things you'd like to achieve in the future.

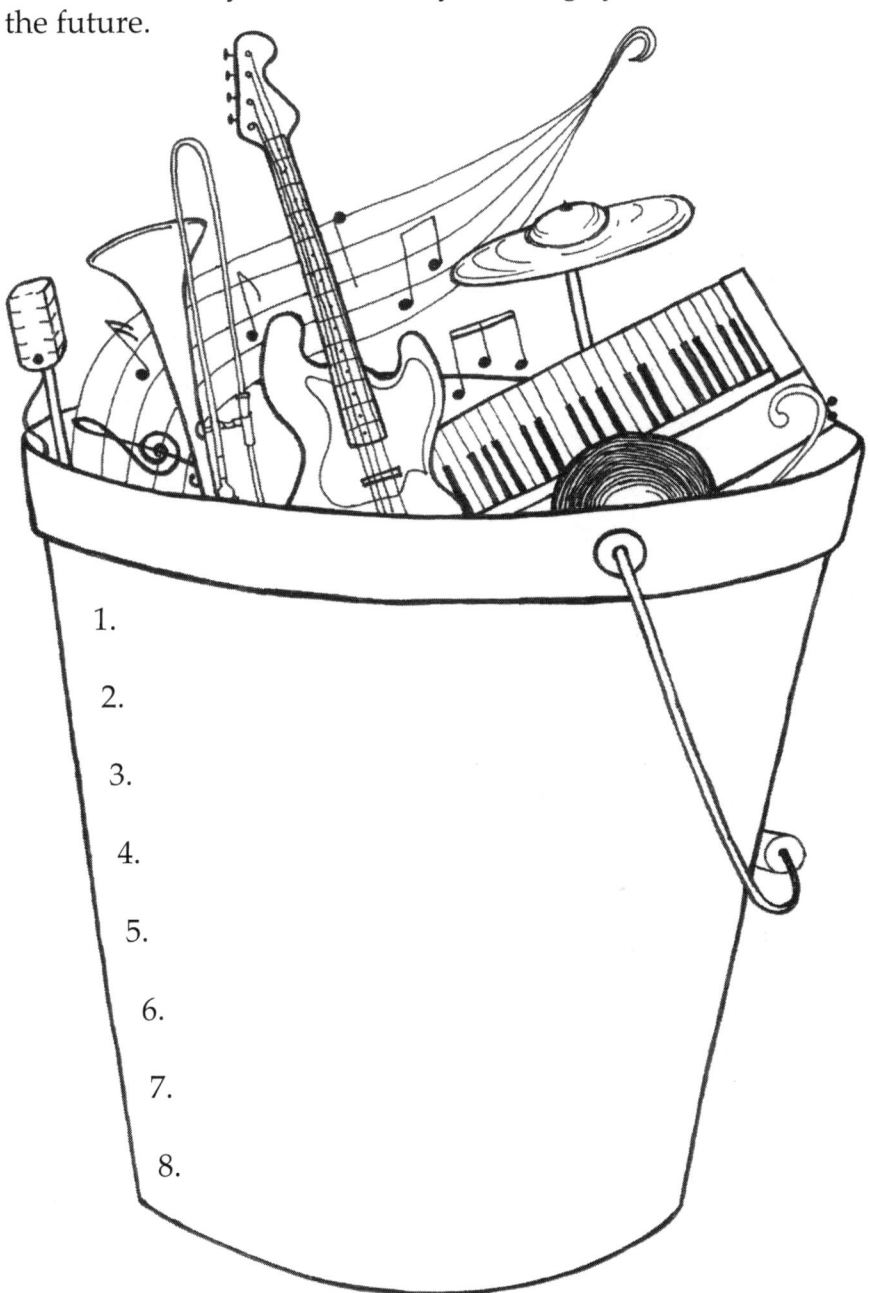

1.
2.
3.
4.
5.
6.
7.
8.

Natural sounds I like to hear

Music that boosts my creativity

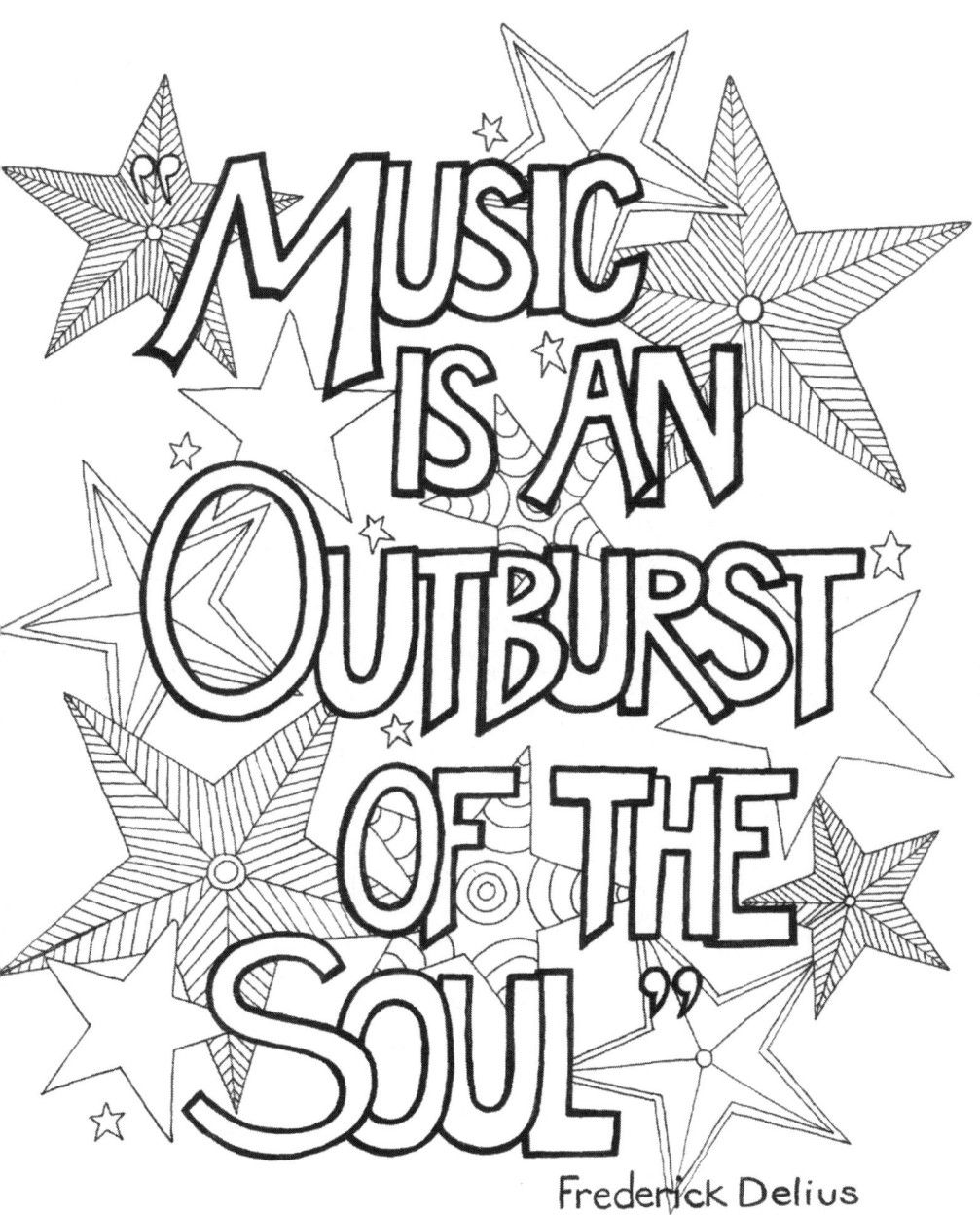

Music that distracts me from unpleasant thoughts

Music that I would like played at my funeral

MEMORY PAGE: Use this page to record music that is are important to you now or in future

My two favourites from 'MY FUTURE' are:

1.

2.

Add these to your playlist on Page 52

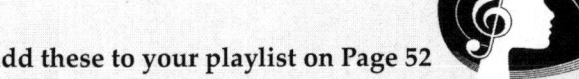

MY DISLIKES

Music genres that I dislike

Particular songs or pieces of music that I dislike

Sounds that I dislike

Particular songs or pieces of music that I find upsetting

Sounds that I find upsetting

MY SOUNDTRACK TO MY LIFE PLAYLIST
Record your favourite songs from each section here in your playlist

1.

2.

3.

4.

5.

6.

7.

8.

9.

10.

11.

12.

Practical Application of 'Soundtrack to My Life'

Once the toolkit has been completed and the tracks of greatest significance have been chosen it is possible to apply the music in practical and therapeutic ways. For this to be most effective it is important to record the reasons why a particular song has been chosen on the memories page.

For example, if you know that a visit to the hospital can be upsetting, identify the songs from the toolkit that have the most relaxing and soothing impact and play these during the visit. Hearing these familiar and comforting songs will help to lessen the anxiety and divert the listener away from the distressing and anxious thoughts.

Similarly, if someone is disorientated and unsure of where they are or who they are with, try using those songs that have been chosen to reconnect with familiar and reassuring aspects of the past e.g. those related to occupation, family or events. Hearing these songs can reconnect the person to those people and places that give comfort and reassurance.

Even creating the **'Soundtrack to My Life'** is of therapeutic value to family and friends, those who may find visits at home or a care home emotionally difficult. Supporting a loved one to collect music and recording it in the toolkit is a useful way to spend a visit. We all value feeling useful, and so supporting others in a person centred way is truly meaningful.

Technology

Your **'Soundtrack to My Life'** toolkit enables you to have a comprehensive playlist of significant music for yourself or an individual. Accessing that music is the most important part of the process.

Music is becoming cheaper and more accessible using technology. There are several ways to use technology to listen to the music directly allowing you to listen wherever and whenever you wish.

Examples of places to access music online include:
- YouTube
- Spotify
- iTunes
- Apple Music
- Amazon Music

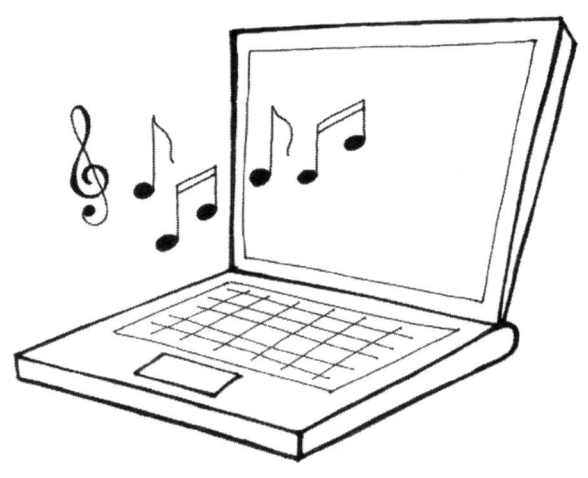

Existing Collections

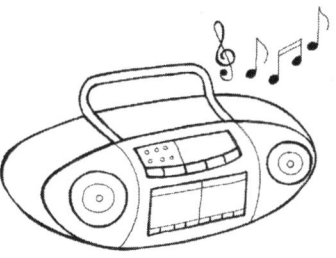

You may already have CDs, records or cassettes that include their significant music and will enable them to access their music.

It is important that you have the right equipment to be able play your music. Using your existing player could be the easiest option as you may already have a full understanding of how to use it. Whatever is the easiest option for you is best but you may want to consider whether that option is portable should you wish to use music outside of your home. You may want to create a CD or MP3 collection of your **'Soundtrack to My Life'** that you can use with a portable device and headphones when not at home. Information on how to create an MP3 playlist or CD are later in this section.

Choosing the Right Device

You must tailor the choice of device to you, the person who will be using it. Think about your ability, for example, if you can use a remote control for a television you may be able to use a device such as tablet, MP3 player etc. Consider size, shape and functionality of a device as well as when and where you may wish to use it. For example, will it be portable if you are away from home, on holiday or visiting family.

Headphones
Equipment such as headphones can create a personalised listening experience if you enjoy using them. Headphones can help to fix your attention on your own playlist when you are in a public room surrounded by other people and competing sounds – or simply if you have difficulty in concentrating.

About the Author

John has spent over 35 years as a provider of health and social care in both the public and private sectors, This includes running his own domiciliary care business. John also cared for his own father who had dementia. As a talented musician he combined his experience of caring and music to create 'Soundtrack to My Life', a music book for people with dementia. In 2012 it won a national care award for innovation.

John, together with his wife Hazel, founded the charity 'musicworks' to support music and musicians in 1995. They support 'Music in Care' projects such as 'Soundtrack to My Life' through a variety of fundraising activities.

In 2012 he established JoCo Learning & Development to develop and deliver 'Soundtrack' training for health and social care staff. John is a passionate believer that high quality care is a right and not a privilege.

If you have been inspired by the content and approach of this book you may also be interested in the other publications in the **'Music in Care'** series.
- **'Soundtrack to My Life'** for people with memory loss conditions including dementia.
- **'My Music Oasis'** for carers either professionally or caring for family members.
- **'My Story in Music'** for people with life-limiting conditions or at end of life.
- **'Music is Medicine'** for people undergoing long term medical treatment.
- **'My Journey in Music'** for young people and those with Asperger's Syndrome and Autism (with Luke Fiddes)

If you wish to further your knowledge and understanding of 'Music in Care' practice, educational programmes are available from JoCo Learning & Development.

About JoCo Learning & Development Ltd.

JoCo provides a range of health & social care training and consultancy services.

Recognising that musical practice skills of frontline staff are generally ignored, they have developed 'Soundtrack to My Life' training. This is a fun and interactive course for healthcare and social care professionals, activity coordinators and musicians to explore the power and use of personalised music in dementia care. 'Soundtrack to My Life' is a programme for every one, whether you have musical skills or none at all.

For more information about 'Soundtrack to My Life', 'Music in Care' or other health and social care training, visit their website.

www.joco.gb.net

About **musicworks**

Music is central to our experience of the world around us. It is a primary source of the way we experience, understand and interpret the world in which we live. It is one of the core experiences that define us, unite us and enrich us.

musicworks *exists to promote all forms of music by encouraging, recognising and showcasing musicians work to help them reach a wider audience.*

As believers in the power of music we are proud to support **'Music in Care'**.

www.musicworksnet.co.uk